THE ENERQI CONNECTION

THE ENERQI CONNECTION

DEMYSTIFYING ACUPUNCTURE

Sheri Laine
L.Ac. DIPLOMATE Ac.

with Tiffany Strause

iUniverse, Inc.
New York Lincoln Shanghai

THE ENERQI CONNECTION
DEMYSTIFYING ACUPUNCTURE

iUniverse books may be ordered through booksellers or by contacting:

iUniverse
2021 Pine Lake Road, Suite 100
Lincoln, NE 68512
www.iuniverse.com
1-800-Authors (1-800-288-4677)

The information, ideas, and suggestions in this book are not intended as a substitute for professional medical advice. Before following any suggestions contained in this book, you should consult your personal physician. Neither the author nor the publisher shall be liable or responsible for any loss or damage allegedly arising as a consequence of your use or application of any information or suggestions in this book.

ISBN-13: 978-0-595-41555-7 (pbk)
ISBN-13: 978-0-595-85902-3 (ebk)
ISBN-10: 0-595-41555-5 (pbk)
ISBN-10: 0-595-85902-X (ebk)

Printed in the United States of America

Contents

Acknowledgments

It has been my dream for nearly two decades to write a primer about Oriental medicine. Thank you, thank you, thank you to my many friends, family, colleagues, and patients for supporting me in realizing my dream. Thank you, Rose, for listening to my ideas and thoughts and still acting interested, if not amused. My Darling, you have been a reliable well source of never-ending inspiration, joy, and love. Angie, how wonderful to work with you, and how lovely to see the beautiful young women you and Amber have become. xoxo.

Tiffany, this project could never have been realized without your inner strength, savvy, and computer brilliance. Many, many, many thanks and much love. I have been very fortunate to have some brilliant and accomplished coaches and mentors in my life. Richard, Barney, Brian, Robert, Charlie, Jeffie, Pete, and Sean: I honor you all. Thank you for letting me draft off your seasoned insights. My patients deserve much credit for their honesty, trust, and faith in me. My heartfelt gratitude to all of you who demonstrate *patience* while I get to continue in practice.

To my beloved Chinese master, Dr. Richard Teh-Fu Tan "Kam pi," thank you for teaching me the meaning of true wisdom and guiding me to the heart and soul of Chinese medicine. *Namaste, Sheri.*

Preface

Traditionally, Chinese medicine is passed down from father to son, or master to apprentice. A Chinese medicine master is both a teacher and a doctor who has practiced for many years. Masters demonstrate skill, intellect, and infinite wisdom, perfecting their technique and style in diagnosis, formulation, and treatment. They constantly reach for and achieve powerful levels of excellence, while earning the respect and admiration of their peers, students, and patients. When a master chooses a student, the decision is not taken lightly, as it is a relationship and commitment that spans a lifetime. My Chinese master, Dr. Richard "Teh-Fu" Tan, carefully chose me to be his apprentice to study Chinese ancestral secrets.

He interviewed me over the course of many meetings, during which he quizzed me intensely on a whole range of things including who my patients were, what their symptoms were, what acupuncture points I chose and why, and what my herbal formulation plans and nutritional evaluations were. He wanted to know what their physical and mental responses were and what I planned for my next treatments. It was like the Inquisition! He threw out herbal formulations in Chinese and asked me if I would consider using them instead of my intended choices. Of course, some of them were the wrong formulas, and I would have to tell him the right ones, in *Chinese!*

This process took almost a year. Once he had made the decision to take me on as his student, he invited me to his favorite Chinese restaurant for an elaborate fish banquet to celebrate the beginning of our work together.

I began studying with him over thirteen years ago after practicing acupuncture in my own private clinic for four years. Once Dr. Tan deemed me a serious and deserving student, he opened up and shared with me the most amazing stories, treatment strategies, and "secret" herbal formulations. Some of these treatment strategies came from his own brilliant calculations while others were handed down from generations past—from his great-great-grandfather who was a physician to many governors in China.

Dr. Tan teaches in both Chinese and English, which can make it hard to figure out exactly what is going on some of the time! For the first year, I was not allowed to ask questions of any kind. My job was simply to observe his treatment techniques, chart patients' progress, clean rooms, answer the phones, make appointments, and handle payments at the front desk. While much of my time in the clinic felt like "slave labor" (think *Karate Kid*), I spent as much time as possible at his elbow in the treatment rooms and in the herbal pharmacy, watching him treat his patients and prepare the herbal formulations. The knowledge I gained was invaluable.

In China, doctors often see and treat ten to twenty-five patients together in the same room or down long hallways, talking openly about physical maladies without any thought to privacy. My teacher Dr. Tan would treat his patients similarly, often seeing up to forty-five patients in my one four-hour weekly shift. Watching him in his clinic and listening to how he answered his patients' and students' questions has most certainly made me a wiser doctor, if not a better analytical thinker. More importantly, he showed me, time and again, what most of us want and need to know when it comes to Oriental medicine.

I wrote this book because I find that most people interested in acupuncture and Oriental medicine have similar questions. Much of the information that is available on acupuncture is confusing, even to me sometimes, and I have been practicing acupuncture for over seventeen years. I've found that there is an overwhelming need for Oriental medicine in our society.

Whether you are looking to lose weight, become balanced, stay healthy, or are just curious, Oriental medicine may provide you with the answers or cure you have been looking for.

Introduction—It's All About Balance

The Chinese first became aware of the principles of acupuncture over five thousand years ago when warriors discovered that certain physical maladies began to improve after receiving puncture wounds from sword fights. Chinese physicians began to take note of the correlations between puncture sites and improved health. They theorized that Qi (pronounced "chee") is the energy or life force that circulates throughout the body, carrying with it our body's blood and oxygen, ensuring healthy functioning of all the bodily systems, organs, and cells. By puncturing the body in specific places, they found they were able to stimulate the body's Qi to heal itself.

President Richard Nixon is credited with bringing acupuncture to America as a new modality of medicine in the 1970s. It is no surprise that what is old is now new again in this cycle of life. Just as fashion trends resurface, the acupuncture of today is based on the premises of ancient times but is carried out in a new way.

In a series of recent studies using ultrasound, scientists have found evidence that "meridians," or energy channels, lie along sheets of connective tissue that surround the organs of the body. The studies found that 80 percent of the acupuncture points correlate with major connective tissue planes found along the meridians. Studies show that acupuncture stimulates the hypothalamus and pituitary glands, which help increase the immune function as well as improve one's mental state. Acupuncture acts on these brain structures to help control the appetite and food cravings. Doctors now routinely prescribe acupuncture for pain management and substance addictions. Acupuncture lowers levels of neurotransmitters, such as norepinephrine and dopamine, which are often elevated in people who experience stress and pain.

Clinical depression is often linked to chronic pain sufferers who feel as though they cannot break the cycle of pain. Acupuncture helps both pain and depression by releasing endorphins and serotonin, which enhance the body's ability to heal itself. The effects of acupuncture have been shown in studies employing brain scans. The scans showed decreased activity in the limbic system, the area that controls emotions. Many acupuncture patients report experiencing a deeper awareness of self and greater capacity for enjoyment and creativity. When patients with addictive challenges are able to stabilize their emotions, they reduce the nervous and repetitive behaviors that feed their unfulfilled emotional needs.

Acupuncturists use needles and their electromagnetic properties to release, charge, and balance or convert Qi, or life force energy, allowing revitalized, changed energy to flow into the body. Needles used during an acupuncture treatment are metal and therefore conduct their own invisible electromagnetic energy field. When we insert acupuncture needles along strategic points in the body called "acupoints," the meeting of the needles and the body's electromagnetic force fields balance the body's entire energy field. We add energy or Qi where it may be lacking or blocked or take away excess Qi where it may be overstimulated. By placing the needles accurately in the body along the meridians, we can strengthen weaknesses, sedate excesses, warm or cool the body, or disperse stagnation to once again allow a healthy flow of energy.

Acupuncture is gaining in popularity because many feel that Western medicine does not fully address our health, weight, and wellness needs, or that certain Western medicine methodologies are too invasive and carry lasting or uncomfortable side effects. These people, like you, are searching for alternatives to fill that gap. Increasingly, Americans are turning to acupuncture to proactively maintain their health. They are finding relief in the fastest growing modality of health care treatment in America, with over 8.2 million Americans turning to acupuncture today. Organizations such as the National Institute of Health (NIH) and the World Health Organization (WHO) have studied acupuncture and its effects and recognize its power to treat a wide variety of conditions. Evidence of its efficacy is growing; studies using brain scans and ultrasound have demonstrated that acupuncture creates direct, measurable, positive effects on the body. A study at the University of California, Irvine, showed, using MRI (functional magnetic resonance imaging), that the visual cortex in the brain was activated when scientists inserted needles along acupoints on the foot that are responsible for vision.

In Western medicine, it is common to treat illness after the fact rather than promoting balance and wellness to prevent illness from occurring in the first place. Too many people wait until a disease has taken hold in their body, even though they know they feel "off balance." The risk of waiting is a weakening of the immune system or changes in the metabolism. When the immune system or metabolism is affected, disease, weight gain, or weight loss are the result. Many patients fall into the category of "not sick, but not really well." They see traditional medical doctors for a myriad of medical challenges but leave with prescriptions to treat *symptoms* instead of solutions for the root cause of their health challenges. Many doctors are not aware of the benefits of acupuncture because they lack training and exposure to Chinese medicine and are therefore hesitant to refer patients to Chinese medical doctors.

In essence, Chinese medicine focuses on balance and wellness, which helps to prevent illness and lifestyle imbalances. Acupuncture also provides a boost to your body's recuperative powers and your metabolism, enabling you to recover your health quickly. By using acupuncture, you will find that it truly is a wonderful and effective medical approach that empowers your body to heal itself. You can expect to feel better while learning what makes your body feel healthier, stronger, and more balanced.

Although acupuncture has no religious affiliations, many experience a deeper spiritual awareness from its profound relaxing effects on the nervous system. Along with the unique calming effects from a treatment, come the ability and the desire to go deeper within. Cloudy questions become clearer, resulting in answers. Where there was once mental inability, there is newfound clarity, enhanced emotional ability, and sustained willpower.

This book intends to help the reader achieve a better understanding of the practice of acupuncture and the concepts of our body's energy and the energy that surrounds us in the world. This knowledge will allow you to be an informed consumer, better able to participate in your own healing process or health maintenance. I came up with a simple mnemonic device to remind my patients about maintaining balance in their lives; maybe it will help you too. I call it the LAINE system, which stands for Learn, Align, Inform, Natural, Energy. Reading this book will help you to Learn About Incredible Natural Energy and how it can change your life. It is my sincere wish that you will be inspired to experience acupuncture and embrace its profound effects in your life. You are about to embark on a new pathway, exploring energy and how it works in our lives.

In December of 1999, I learned that I had chronic myelogenous leukemia (CML). After the initial shock and learning that I had no acceptable donor for a bone marrow transplant, I started on a course of therapy with interferon alpha. After eighteen months of daily injections, I was very depressed and extremely tired. I had also contracted peripheral neuropathy, due to those treatments, in my feet. This condition made walking very painful. My oncologist indicated that there was very little that he could do for the condition other than take me off the medication. Since that was an unacceptable option, I had to look for alternatives. After searching the Internet and speaking with other CML patients, I learned that acupuncture might be an effective alternative treatment for the peripheral neuropathy. I was very skeptical of this therapeutic approach since I am a doctor in the pharmaceutical field. However, out of desperation, I started on a course of acupuncture therapy. After several months of massage and acupuncture treatments, I started to feel the pain abate. Today, I am able to walk without pain, and I feel more alive than ever. I also learned that Western medical science does not have all of the answers and that acupuncture therapy should be used in a synergistic approach to the treatment of pain.

—K.G., male, late fifties

LEARN

Chapter 1—Is Acupuncture for Me?

If I always do what I've always done, I'll always get what I've always got.
—Ross Quinn

Let's find out whether your life is in balance. Read through the following questions as you think about your life. When you're finished, count the number of your A, B, and C answers. Then see the key below to find out how balanced you are and how acupuncture can help you.

1. When I wake, I feel

    A. refreshed and ready to start my day.

    B. sluggish, but after some caffeine I'm raring to go.

    C. dead tired and already thinking about my afternoon nap.

2. I drink

    A. four to six glasses of room temperature water or warm herbal tea a day.

    B. only the bottle of water I keep in the car.

    C. only Diet Coke or iced tea.

3. I have a bowel movement at least once a day, usually within 25–45 minutes of waking:

    A. Absolutely!

    B. Some days are better than others.

C. I am often constipated.

4. I exercise regularly (i.e., three to five times a week for 25 to 75 minutes each time):

    A. Yes, it's an important part of my life.

    B. If I have the time I will.

    C. Never, I hate it.

5. My diet includes plenty of fresh seasonal fruits and vegetables:

    A. Yes, I love eating healthy and will go out of my way to do so.

    B. I try to be conscientious, but I usually just grab whatever is around when I am hungry.

    C. Does it count if it comes out of a can or the freezer?

6. I consider myself a moderate social drinker:

    A. I drink under seven alcoholic beverages a week (and not all in one night).

    B. When I am in a social setting, it's easy to get carried away.

    C. Who's counting anyway?

7. I have a job that allows me to be my creative best, and I enjoy myself there:

    A. Yes, I love my work.

    B. I'm comfortable in my job but often fantasize about moving on.

    C. C. I dread going to work every day.

8. I have a fun, supportive, stimulating social circle of friends that inspire me to be and do my very best:

   A. Yes, my friends are warm and supportive.

   B. My friends are OK, but I am often left feeling dissatisfied.

   C. No, my friends are difficult and often a source of stress.

9. My romantic and sexual needs are met, or at least I am getting closer to having them met through effective communication:

   A. Yes, although I do have the usual ups and downs.

   B. I have had my disappointments, but there is always hope.

   C. I don't even know what I want; I'm too busy to take the time to figure it out.

10. Outside of work

    A. I make time to pursue my hobbies.

    B. I seem to run a lot of errands and do a lot of chores.

    C. I watch TV and surf the web.

11. To me, inner reflection means

    A. making time to go within and get quiet.

    B. trying to stop my thoughts.

    C. figuring out what I am going to have for dinner.

12. My body aches:

    A. Rarely. I am mostly free from nagging aches.

    B. Often.

    C. Always. It seems I always have a little ache somewhere.

13. On the whole, my life is
    A. Happy.
    B. generally OK.
    C. in need of help.
14. I have a few extra pounds to lose:
    A. Not at all.
    B. On and off throughout my life.
    C. Don't ask, don't tell!

If you answered A to ten or more, you are a happy, fulfilled, balanced human being. Your healthy lifestyle is a priority for you and it shows! You enjoy your work pursuits and understand the value of strong, evolving relationships with others. Acupuncture will help you maintain balance in your life.

If you answered B to eight or more, you may feel like you ride shotgun through life. While life is generally OK and you don't have too many complaints, you know that you are capable of creating more for yourself. Acupuncture will help you to improve your life by putting *you* back in the driver's seat, empowering you to be healthier and happier while improving your energy.

If you answered C to five or more, you feel more "off" than "on." You *know* it is time to make a change! You have nothing to lose and everything to gain. The sky is the limit for what you can create if you take the time to explore who you are, what you want, and what you truly value. Acupuncture will help you to begin your inner journey now!

Congratulations! You are on the right track to a strong, healthy, balanced life. Only you have the power to create true balance in your life. Change is truly the only constant thing in life, and once you have achieved balance, you will be open and welcome to change and growth. This is what Qi energy is all about!

"I have suffered with sinus problems since I was a teenager. I was unaware of what my condition was and just thought I had more colds than most people. When I was in my 20s, I began relying on nasal sprays and over-the-counter decongestants to enable me to breathe through my nose instead of my mouth. In my 30s, I started getting sinus infections, which were extremely painful, and began using doctor-prescribed antibiotics and steroid medications to relieve my symptoms. I continued with these treatments until my mid-50s when a friend suggested I try acupuncture. I noticed a significant difference within several weeks. I was breathing well and had far fewer headaches. I have continued treatment for the past six years and have not had a sinus infection or used a nasal spray in that time. It has truly changed my quality of life for the better.

I initially started acupuncture treatments for my sinus problems, but it has helped me with other health issues as well. It gave me extra strength to get through breast cancer treatment and some difficult emotional times. These latter benefits I attribute directly to my particular acupuncturist who in addition to her skill as an acupuncturist is a good listener who gives sage council."

—*C.B., female, early 60s*

Chapter 2—Qi: What Is It, and How Does It Work?

Learning is weightless, a treasure you can always carry easily.
—Chinese proverb

Acupuncture serves to balance Qi (your life force or vital energy), which circulates in and around all of us. Look around you at your environment. How does it make you feel? Everything carries with it its own energetic, vibrating force field called Qi. Notice how you feel when you are in the mountains or by the sea, looking up at the blue or gray skies and smelling the air that circulates around you. After spending time outside in nature, most of us feel charged, lifted, connected, and changed. This feeling of harmony is from the energy your body has absorbed from the environment.

How about when you walk into a clean, bright, thoughtfully decorated home or restaurant? Don't you notice it makes you feel good? Compare that feeling to walking into a dark, dingy, dirty establishment; most of us can't wait to get out of there. It has a weird vibration, an "ick" factor. We have all felt this "ick" factor and are relieved to be away from it. When you are in tune with your body, it is in tune with the environment, and you are much more sensitive to, and in touch with, other people and your surroundings.

Yin and Yang

The Chinese use the concept of opposite, interdependent energies to highlight the necessity of balance. The warmth of summer surrenders to the coolness of autumn and later to the coldness of winter. The cycle continues as the shorter, colder, darker days give way to the longer, lighter days of spring and continues on with warmth again in the summer. The night always becomes the day, and the day always becomes the night. Like day and night, yin and yang (say "yahng") are opposites that are intertwined. One always balances the other.

Yin is considered the white, internal, feminine, earthy, wet, cool, intuitive, contemplative energy. Yang is the black, external, masculine, the endless skies, dry, hot, action-oriented energy. We all have a unique combination of yin/yang Qi energy in our bodies. This combination can change daily based on our lifestyle choices. We feel yin energy when we don't want to get out of bed in the morning, and we feel yang energy when, before the alarm, we are wide awake and ready to start our day.

Constitutional Strength and Qi

We are all born with a certain amount of Qi, which is our body's constitutional strength and the vital force inherent in all things. Think of Qi as your body's root system, a system that is always in place to feed and nourish you, especially if you have taken good care of it. This root strength, our Qi, can be maintained and strengthened through a balanced lifestyle. Acupuncture and herbal medicines are a powerful way to balance your lifestyle and enhance your Qi. This system carries our physical, mental, and spiritual power within it, and it is what energetically charges us.

We experience our Qi in terms of our energy levels. Our Qi changes based on how we take care of ourselves, what we think about, and the lifestyle choices we make. I have coined a term for this that I call "EnerQi" (ener-chee). We all know how bad we feel when we've been caught off balance and have not been good to ourselves. Not being good to ourselves looks like: poor dietary choices, abuse of foods and libations, negative or unproductive thinking and or communications, lack of sufficient sleep and exercise, etc. The longer we remain off balance the worse we usually feel. By being balanced, your energetic frequency will be raised to a much higher level, making you feel stronger and more alive than ever before. As you begin to experience the power of your enhanced enerQi, you will find there really is no going back. You simply will feel too good and too in touch with your true powerful inner self. The more you focus on the principles of balance in life, the more in touch you will be with your body's enerQi and the better you will become at fine-tuning your body's enerQi voltage with ease.

We are also born with another very important substance called "Jing essence." We inherit Jing essence from our parents at birth. This essence, which is another power within us, determines our constitutional strength, the vitality we are born with. Unlike Qi, Jing essence is much more difficult to strengthen. Jing essence is stored in the kidneys, whereas Qi is stored throughout the body. Unfortunately, once our Jing essence is gone, the candle goes out, and life has come to an end.

While we interact with a lot of people everyday, once in a while you feel you "connect" with someone. We have all heard of animal magnetism, an attraction that we cannot explain or rationalize, that inexplicably draws us to a complete stranger, be it a member of the same or opposite sex. We feel compelled to talk with them; they interest us. I believe that powerful connection is due to Qi energy. We are attracted to that particular vibration because it connects and balances with our own energy. Qi expresses itself as a strong energy field that becomes stronger when we are balanced. By using acupuncture to balance your enerQi, you will feel healthier, happier, more relaxed, and fulfilled. You will also have the enhanced ability to absorb the positive Qi vibrations from the world around you. You will find that your body just works better.

Think of an acupuncture treatment the same way you think of a tune-up for your car. It always has more get-up-and-go after a service! You will see the positive magnetic effects of your amplified enerQi as you become more balanced. People will naturally gravitate to you when your enerQi is pulsating with health, creativity, and vitality. When you are balanced, you are happy and empowered to have the life you want, the body you want, the job you want, and the relationships you want. These positive aspects of life are attracted to your energetic force field, creating pulsating magnetic Qi power that manifests itself powerfully.

Meridians and Qi

The Chinese believe that our bodies are lined with crisscrossing internal and external invisible pulsating energy fields called meridians, which are thought to be electromagnetic. Your body's Qi, blood, and oxygen charge them. Our Qi travels along these meridians, forming channels to move and distribute life force up, down, in, and around the entire body. These meridians cover us like loosely wrapped mummies in gauze and connect to our blood, capillaries, muscles, tendons, joints, bones, internal organs, genitals, limbs, brain, limbic system, eyes, ears, nose, teeth, and mouth. When it comes to the body's energy, twelve of these fields are called the main meridians, and two are the master meridians. For the purposes of this discussion, we will focus only on these fourteen meridians.

One of these master meridians represent the feminine aspect of our energy, the other represents the masculine. In the Oriental medical mind, when Qi is vital and flowing strongly throughout the body, our blood supply is enriched and oxygenated, which in turn supplies the organs with much needed vitality and health. When our Qi becomes blocked or stagnant, the result, in principle, is an excess or deficiency in Qi, blood, or oxygen in our bodies, which increases or decreases the activity of our bodily systems. Our Qi can become blocked for a variety of reasons, including but not limited to poor nutrition, injury, lack of sleep, stress, mental outlook on life, excessive dampness, cold, or heat.

Stagnation and Qi

Stagnation, or blocked Qi, is a buzzword in Chinese medicine. The Chinese consider stagnation to be one of our body's "great evil entities." Unfortunately, a lot of people suffer from stagnation. There are five different kinds of stagnation: food, fluid, cold, Qi, and blood. Any one of these can cause an inflammatory condition.

Think of a pool of crystal-clear blue moving water. In order for the water in the pool to stay clean and free of harmful bacteria, it needs the movement from the current of the wind or a filtering system to aid in circulation. This current circulates the water, keeps it clean, and keeps the energy contained there moving freely. When the water is still, with no movement, over time it becomes a dirty, smelly breeding ground for insects, disease, and bacteria, which cause inflammation; we call this an "evil entity." Herein lies the reason why it is so important for us to give our bodies the proper mental, spiritual, nutritional, and physical care. When our Qi becomes blocked, the movement that is needed for circulation and oxygenation (which makes us and keeps us strong, vibrant, and healthy) is not available to nourish our bodies properly.

Our immune system, energy levels, weight, and general overall happiness and wellness are strong indicators of how balanced our Qi is. How well is your immune system protecting you? Imbalanced Qi can lead to pain, disease, and lethargy. A skilled acupuncturist can diagnose where an imbalance is and correct it by inserting needles into acupoints along meridians. Each acupoint on our body (and there are an infinite number of them to choose from) corresponds to a particular organ or systemic function. Chinese doctors believe that the body's meridians are electromagnetic and that each one has its own energetic Qi vibration along these meridians. These meridians serve as a grid for us to look for and distribute enerQi, blood, and oxygen within the limbic systems, organs, tendons, ligaments, nerves, and muscles by using pressure or puncture techniques. By restoring the balance of our body's natural electromagnetic energy, the body can heal itself and function properly.

Qi as a River

A useful analogy to help explain the concept of Qi and meridians is to imagine that your body's internal workings are a network of streams and estuaries of clean, clear water. Sticks, stones, leaves, or large rocks can get in the way of the flow of this water. These obstructions are our physical and mental imbalances, our life's travails, the bumps and bruises, hurts, and misunderstandings we experience along the way. A weakened immune system, constant emotional upheavals in our lives, weight challenges, restless or sleepless nights, ongoing fatigue and lethargy, or a never-ending litany of aches and pains are our body's way of telling us it has distress from the dis-ease we are experiencing within. It may be a matter of lifestyle choices, which proper diet, exercise, and sleep may remedy. However, once obstructed, the water (or Qi) is forced to take another pathway down the stream by going around the rocks or under the leaves. The water still makes its way down the stream, but not in the most effective or efficient manner. At times, not enough water is coursing through the stream; at other times too much water causes flooding. Acupuncture needles serve as a sweeping branch to brush the accumulated debris away and allow the water to continue in a smooth and timely flow.

I was dealing with a sciatic nerve injury for over eight months, which caused me a great amount of pain in my right leg and back. I had tried everything from my traditional medical doctor, to a chiropractor, to a physical therapist without achieving much relief from my pain. My older sister, who had successfully quit smoking by using acupuncture, suggested I try it. Although I was unconvinced, I had exhausted all other options. My first visit was very thorough, as we discussed not only my injury, but also my overall health and habits. We spent much more time talking than any Western doctor had ever spent with me. After our initial consultation, I learned we would be treating my injury as well as my overall health. That was a first for me! The treatments were easy and relaxing. After several months, I am 98 percent better and am able to proceed pain free in my normal, everyday life. I would recommend acupuncture to anyone who wants an alternative to a scalpel or drugs and wants to be healed by their body's own energy. Acupuncture must be effective, why else would it be in practice for over five thousand years!

—P.L., fifty-one-year-old male

Chapter 3—Why Should I Pay Someone to Stick Me with Needles?

Life belongs to the living, and he who lives must be prepared for changes.

—Goethe

Many people try acupuncture when they have exhausted all contemporary Western medical options. Often patients are given the choice of drastic surgery, more drugs, or continued pain and suffering because nothing further can be done for them. They are desperate and ready to try something new. Many of my patients fall into the "not sick, but not well" category. They fall through the cracks of Western medicine, and often acupuncture can help.

In my practice, I have successfully treated with acupuncture:

- Weight challenges: weight gain, weight loss, obesity, anorexia, bulimia
- Internal organs: stomach digestion, nausea, IBS, colitis, ulcers, constipation problems, hypoglycemia, hemorrhoids, stroke, Bell's palsy, trigeminal neuralgia, cerebral palsy, polio, chronic fatigue
- Hay fever and allergies (seasonal and food related)
- External systems: addictions (prescription pain medication, recreational drug abuse, food, alcohol), hangovers
- Self-development and growth
- Dermatological issues: eczema, psoriasis, acne, shingles, herpes (oral and genital), hair loss, edema, hives
- Muscles, tendons, ligaments, nerves: fibromyalgia, arthritis, back pain (upper, middle, low), sciatica, neck pain, shoulder pain (including frozen shoulder syndrome), tendonitis, stiff neck, bursitis, carpal tunnel syndrome, TMJ, tennis elbow
- Sports injuries: sprains and strains
- Emotional/mental pain: panic attacks, anxiety, depression, mood disorders, ADD and ADHD, sleep disorders
- Stress: high or low blood pressure, headaches

- Ears, eyes, nose and throat: infections, colds, flu, bronchitis, pneumonia, ear aches, sore throat, sinusitis, asthma, ringing in ear (high or low), deafness
- OB/GYN: premenstrual syndrome, amenorrhea, cramping, infertility, menopause symptoms, hot flashing, night sweats, flooding (menorraghia), pelvic inflammatory disease, ovarian cysts
- Pregnancy: morning sickness, breech presentation before delivery, inducement of labor, lactation insufficiency, milk fever
- Seasickness, motion sickness
- Meneres disease, vertigo
- Presurgical care and postsurgical care
- Sexual dysfunction (male or female)

While most of the health issues listed are not going to prevent you from living your day-to-day life, they are annoying enough to make living life more difficult. Some of these imbalances are certainly more challenging than others; however, I have been able to see positive changes in all of my patients regardless of severity of symptoms.

Individuals who have incurable autoimmune disorders often use acupuncture to support their immune system function. In my practice, I have also treated patients with the following:

- AIDS
- Cancer
- Diabetes
- Hepatitis
- Lupus

- Lyme disease
- MS
- Parkinsonism and Parkinson disease
- Other serious autoimmune disorders

Run, don't walk (limp if you must!), to your acupuncturist if you are bruised, swollen, sick, inflamed, in pain, or otherwise under the weather. The sooner you get yourself there, the faster your recovery!

Four years ago when I first tried acupuncture, I had a host of health issues. I was suffering from depression, had a rash that covered my arms, legs, and torso, in addition to irregular heartbeats, fatigue, and headaches. None of the physicians I had seen in the past seven years could tell me what I had or help me. After my first meeting with Sheri, she suspected that one of my problems was food allergies. She put me on a restricted diet, and within weeks, I felt better. We also discovered that I have an autoimmune disease. With acupuncture treatments, my rash began to disappear, and my immune system is a lot more stable. Acupuncture, herbs, [and] dietary and lifestyle modifications changed my outlook, and I now know I can live a long and healthy life. Words can never express my gratitude. Thank you for helping me!

—D.K., forty-seven-year-old female

ALIGN

Chapter 4—What Qualifies You to Do This, and How Do You Know Where to Put Those Things?

To be successful the first thing to do is fall in love with your work.
—Sr. Mary Lauretta

Getting Educated

Licensed acupuncturists complete an extremely rigorous, comprehensive study program that requires approximately four years, with a full-time commitment after receiving an associate degree. Requirements vary from state to state; check with your local medical examining board for exact regulations. In addition to learning all Western medical sciences, we are trained in traditional Chinese medical sciences, Chinese medical theory, Chinese anatomy (meridian and acupuncture point locations), Chinese philosophical studies, herbal medicine theory and preparation, clinical counseling, and *Tui Nui* (say "twee naw"), a particular Chinese method of massage and bone setting. We must also participate for two years in tai chi and Qi gong (pronounced "chee-gung") exercise classes, which cultivate self-awareness and strengthen Qi within the body. A lot of this information is presented in Chinese, as well as in English—try learning medicine in a completely new language that you can't initially understand, let alone read or pronounce!

From the first semester on, you find out if this work is your life's calling; it is a difficult and all-consuming path. Many students drop like flies after starting their second semester. The dedication required to your study, the constant rote memorization, the never-ending multiple exams, and the time it takes in this pursuit is enormous, humbling, and definitely life altering. For example, we students had to literally strip down in front of our classmates, allowing them to poke, prod, and mark our bodies to learn where to find the acupoints and to practice their palpation and needling techniques.

After the second year and until graduation two years later, we are required to begin treating patients under close supervision in the community clinic or in the local teaching hospitals, working side by side with other medical and acupuncture students. Our teachers could not stress enough the importance of our duty, as doctors, to focus, watch, and observe very carefully the patient's general presentation, coloring, demeanor, gait, and posture. As we complete our training, we see how Chinese medicine differs significantly from the Western view by taking into account the whole being and by incorporating a very careful observance by the doctor.

Let the Scrutiny Begin: The First Visit

The first impression is important and begins as soon as the patient walks up the path to the clinic. In my experience, people show up in one of three modes: warrior mode, prisoner mode, or art-of-life mode.

Warriors are classic Type A's who have difficulty relaxing and shutting down their minds. Prisoners act the victim and are often very weary and afraid. The art-of-life person is more evenly balanced and is a strategic thinker, able to handle challenges they encounter in life easier than most. Diagnosis begins the moment you meet your practitioner and shake hands. When our eyes meet upon introduction, a list of questions begins to form in my mind, such as, what is the shade of the whites of your eyes? How clear are they? Are your irises clear and shiny or cloudy and dull? Is your grip strong or limp like a dead fish? Are your hands clammy or dry? Do you have a distinct odor, and is it sweet, acrid or greasy? Does your skin look appropriate for your age? Is it dewy and glowing or dry, hanging and excessively wrinkled?

People will often be wearing the colors of their diagnosis in the clothing choices they make. In addition, reading the physical characteristics of the face helps determine what type of personality traits you carry with you in the world. The shape of your ears and nostrils are clues to your general Qi strength. The answers to these diagnostic observational questions are indicators of the general yin/yang balances in the body and are an important starting point that determines your course of treatment.

There is a Buddhist saying I often refer to: "If you cannot find the truth right where you are, where do you expect to find it?" It is very important to feel comfortable, confident, and safe with your choice of practitioner in all aspects of medicine. Acupuncture is a holistic approach to health. What this means is that through meaningful conversations during the intake period we will explore together who you are mentally, spiritually, and physically, and how you approach your life. This discovery is the essence of mind-body medicine. Because all of us have different ways of communicating, it is important that you feel comfortable with your practitioner and that his or her communication style works for you. If for any reason you are uncomfortable or find yourself not honestly sharing what really goes on in your life, certainly after several sessions, you may need to find another person to work with. Your energy vibration needs to fit and feel comfortable with that of your practitioner's. If you can't honestly share what you are experiencing or are not ready to at least explore what that is, then you are not well matched with your practitioner or are not ready to be helped.

The Questionnaire

As a new patient, you will be asked to fill out a *very* detailed questionnaire about how your body works and what prior injuries and illnesses you have experienced, in addition to what medications and nutritional supplements you are currently taking. If you have weight issues, you may be asked to keep a 4 to 7 day journal of all the things you eat and drink and to bring that journal to your appointment. This will give your acupuncturist a clearer idea of your habits.

Be prepared to answer a lot of questions, starting at the top of your head and working down to your toes. I will want to know intimate details about what goes in and what comes out, the tastes you crave, the temperature of the foods you eat, what you choose to eat, how much you eat, and when you eat it. How much sleep do you get in an average night? If you have decided to see an acupuncturist for an athletic injury, strain, or sprain, we will not focus on the comprehensive internal medical exam as in depth. Instead, we will want to get you out of pain as soon as possible by increasing circulation of blood and oxygen to the area of the injury. This will help reduce the bruising, swelling, and inflammation. We will pay attention to the internal working of your body, but the first inclination will be to reduce pain.

Other questions will follow, such as:

- Does your meal sit in your stomach, making you feel bloated and sleepy, or do you easily digest your meals and feel energized after eating?
- How do you feel when you wake up, and how are you doing when you lie down to rest at the end of the day?
- Are you a daytime napper?
- At night, what time do you go to sleep, and how well do you sleep? Do you toss and turn or sleep like a rock? Do you have dreams that disturb your sleep?
- Are you generally hot or cold? Does your body temperature respond according to your surroundings?
- Do you sweat or shiver in your sleep?
- What, if anything, hurts? What is the quality of that pain—sharp and stabbing or deep and achy? Are your muscles generally tight and sore?

- What is the time of day or night that you have the most energy?
- How sexually active are you?
- Are you performing as well as you would like to in all physical activity, including sex?

Your communication style says a lot about you, as does your posture and how engaged you are when answering questions. Do you know what it is you need to become more fulfilled? I will be asking myself in this portion of the diagnosis: "Who is this person really?" and "What makes them tick?" A picture is starting to develop for me.

Most people really do know their bodies; they know what is working and what is not working for them in their lives. Freely admitting it is another thing! Talking through symptoms and challenges usually helps people focus on getting in touch with what is wrong and what they need. We partner together by combining your intimate knowledge of you with my insights and knowledge. I need to get to know you to treat you.

As we create your treatment plan, it will be clear at that time how many treatments you will need in order to see the changes we will both be looking for. Everyone is different, and some will need more or less than others. A ballpark estimate will depend on whether your condition is long-term or short-term and what your goals are. Initially, a typical course will include acupuncture treatments once or twice a week, sometimes even three times a week, for about six to twelve weeks. Again, length of time depends on the severity of the symptoms. As your symptoms fade away and you begin to feel in balance, we will both know when it is time to reduce the number of visits.

Say "Ahhh"!

You will then be asked to show your tongue to tell further what is going on inside your body. Yes, stick it all the way out! We will be interested in its size, length, shape, various colors, coating, color of the coating, location of the coating, wetness or dryness of the coating, and any demarcations seen there.

Your tongue tells, quite distinctly, what is going on inside your body; it gives your doctor a very clear reflection of your internal organs. Each organ has a delineated area that mirrors itself on the tongue's surface. The color of your tongue reflects the condition of your blood, Qi, and yin organs. A normal tongue color is light red. Ideally, the tongue should look like a piece of fresh, raw meat. So, if your tongue were for sale at the grocery store, would you buy it? The shape of the tongue reflects the condition of your blood and Qi. Its size mirrors the health or the weakness of these substances. The coating indicates the state of the yang organs, especially the stomach. A normal coating should be thin and light white.

Tap Into This!

We will want to palpate the abdomen, which includes pressing and tapping. The temperature of your body's "Ming Men Fire" can be felt right below the navel. This is an area we look for to be warm, as the degree of warmth felt there is another indicator of how your body's internal engine is performing. You should not be experiencing any kind of pain upon palpation. We will be looking at skin tone, cold, hot, or warm temperature distribution, or any uncommon hardness; we will also notice any unusual pain response to light pressure. Some people have boundaries about being touched, so expect your practitioner to ask permission before palpating your abdomen.

On the Pulse

The next step is to feel the body's pulses. They are located at the outside of each wrist. They can be found by placing three fingers (pointer, index, and ring finger) very gently, one after the other, slightly below the thenar eminence (pad of the thumb) on the lateral or outside part of your wrist. You may notice a very light pressure as the superficial and deeper levels of the pulse qualities are located.

According to Chinese medical theory, we have twelve pulses in total, six yin and six yang. When it comes to the body's energy, the pulses represent the organ activity, which incorporates Western medical concepts of the organs. Here is where the idea of organ systems strongly differs in Chinese theory and concept: organ pulses are divided into two main groups. The yin organs (inner and deeper) hold and store while the yang organs (outer and more superficial) transport and move. There are six pulses on the right side and six pulses on the left side. They are paired in yin/yang partnership, with each set representing one element of nature (Fire, Earth, Metal, Water, and Wood). Each yin/yang pair depends on the other to function as a whole. Remember, yin becomes yang as yang becomes yin, so disharmony in one part of the element usually affects its pair.

The Elements

The Fire element represents the heart (yin) and small intestines (yang)

The Earth element represents the spleen (yin) and stomach (yang)

The Metal element represents the lung (yin) and large intestine (yang)

The Water element represents the kidney (yin) and bladder (yang)

The Wood element represents the liver (yin) and gallbladder (yang)

There is also a deeper principle within the pulses, one of pure yang and one of pure yin, that I will be feeling for in your pulse.

Another set of pulses, which are known as the san jiao or "triple burner," is then located. These "burner" pulses are intermingled with the twelve total pulses. They give further information about the inner workings of breathing, digestion, elimination, and the energy consumption processes within your body. After a quick check of the pedal pulses, which are located at the inside of the ankle, to ascertain heart health, it is also common to check blood pressure, which ideally should be in the 110/75 range.

Gathering More Information about You

If you have had any lab work done, I will want to look at the findings. I will also be interested to know your cholesterol count. If you are over fifty, I'll want to know whether you've had a colonoscopy and the results, as well as the results of your most recent gynecological and breast exam for women and prostate exam for men. If I feel I need more information, I will order more lab work through an independent laboratory or ask that you go through your primary care doctor to request those tests. Using all diagnostic tools, along with the information that has been gathered from you, I can ascertain what your body needs to become more balanced and more powerful.

At last, it is time to enhance your enerQi!

"I decided to try acupuncture because my shoulder was bothering me, and all the normal medicine and even an osteopath using nonmainstream technique was not helping. All the symptoms seemed to return. I needed to try something else. I was also in a period of self-discovery, working on my issues for the first time in my life. Although I had lots of support at my church and great friends, I felt I could make choices I never had before. Trying something new was part of loving myself and taking responsibility for my own health and well-being.

[During] my first session, I was apprehensive because it was something I had never experienced before. When you open yourself up to healing, whether it's the soul, spirit, physical or emotional, one can feel very vulnerable. I found that my acupuncturist's manner and empathy, her ability to differentiate, etc., while connecting to the patient (me in this case) while properly diagnosing and treating, was as important as the treatment.

[During] the second session, I began to really see some effects from the treatment. I felt much more relaxed, I had more energy, and my overall outlook on life improved. Since that time, I have improved, and … my original problem shoulder [has] greatly improved."

—B.L.S., male, late forties

Chapter 5—What's a Session Like, and What Exactly Am I Getting Myself Into?

The mind is like a parachute; it works best when it is open.
—Anonymous

Most acupuncture treatments take place in a private or semiprivate treatment room that is quiet, clean, comfortable, and serene. Usually, the patient lies down or relaxes in a reclining position. It is a good idea to wear loose-fitting and comfortable clothing so that the acupuncturist can access your acupoints easily. At your first treatment, ask to hold and touch the acupuncture needles so you can become more comfortable with them. Most people are surprised by how tiny, flexible, and interesting the needles look—not at all like they had imagined them to be.

All needles are prepackaged, sterilized, single use, and disposable. They are made from high-quality, surgical stainless steel. The thickness of the average Chinese acupuncture needle ranges from 28-44 gauges, and they're from 0.12 mm to 0.35 mm in length. The thinner the gauge of the needle, the less Qi stimulus you will feel upon insertion. Dr. Tan says, "The thinner the needle, the more the treatments!" Some needles have a plastic colored handle on the top that is usually an indication of their size. Some are topped with a copper-, gold-, or silver-colored filigree head. Most acupuncture needles are like fine filaments of silver or gold. Usually, they are very flexible and can bend very easily. The pointed tip is quite small yet very, very sharp. Many people think of a big hypodermic needle coming at them when they hear about acupuncture treatments, but this is not the case at all.

Some practitioners place a metal or plastic tube to lightly press the skin down and insert the needles through the tube. Other practitioners (including myself for the most part) will forgo the tube and just insert the needle very quickly and precisely into the designated area of the body. The decision to use the tube method or the nontube method usually has to do with one's training, not necessarily one's skill. A practitioner who uses a tube has studied more in the traditional Japanese/Korean methods of medicine. The Qi response is slightly less, as is the energetic frequency in the body. The practitioner who uses the "no tube" method has studied the more traditional Chinese methods. Initially, the Qi insertion response is more pronounced, and the energetic frequency is stronger.

The designated needling sites are cleaned with a sterile cotton ball soaked in alcohol or a fresh alcohol swab before insertion. Upon insertion of the needle, you may feel a pinch or the smallest sting, like a rubber band snapping against your skin, or perhaps you'll feel nothing at all. That is normal. The truth is that sometimes for a mere moment there is the smallest amount of discomfort. It should never last for more than a moment. Sometimes a blood vessel will inadvertently be nicked. You may feel a bruising, aching sensation. (If that happens, you might get an instant bruise, which can be treated with immediate pressure applied to the area.) You may see a light bruise develop within hours or a few days after your treatment. It sometimes happens that a nerve will be touched. If that is the case, you will feel an electrical shock sensation that shoots up or down the area where the needle was placed. We'll *both* know when that happens, and I will move the needle immediately. These instances are somewhat common, although we try hard to avoid them! If or when they do happen, there are a few moments of discomfort at most.

In 3 percent of cases, someone will have what we refer to as "needle shock." If you fall into this 3 percent, it means that you will feel faint or actually will faint. Because acupuncture generally requires that you be in a reclining position or lying down, you won't have far to fall. You may experience a clammy, sweaty, dizzy sensation. Your practitioner is right there by your side should this occur and will notice and remedy this situation immediately by taking out your needles. If needed, we will revive you by putting gentle pressure or inserting a needle into one or several points on your body that are specifically for needle shock. A cool cloth, placed on the back of the neck or top of the head, can also help. This phenomenon has happened to me twice in seventeen years of practice. My patients recovered immediately and went on to have wonderful sessions.

For some people, the original complaint is activated by the treatment, and you might experience a day or two of increased pain or symptoms. This is not abnormal. When that subsides, you will begin to feel better. Acupuncturists are also trained in CPR and life resuscitation techniques should there be any other kind of emergencies.

Often, after the initial prick, you may feel pressure or an aching sensation around the needle site. Some practitioners will twist the needles upon insertion or midway through your treatment, or they may adjust the needles by quickly vibrating them up and down. This technique is known as "calling the Qi."

Sometimes, there will be a raised, slightly pink or red ring around the needle insertion point, known as a histamine response. Patients often report a tingly, warm, pulling sensation as well. This is your body's Qi coming up to "greet" the needle's electromagnetic field. At times, you can feel all or none of these sensations, or you may even experience these sensations in areas of your body where there are no needles. Sometimes, one of the needles will begin to buzz and stop, and the next one will buzz and stop, and so on down the line. Sometimes all the needles can be activated at one time and pulsate and/or throb. All patients have their own unique Qi experience as their bodies become balanced. There is no "right" or "wrong" feeling that takes place. Your experience is just that, *your* experience. You should never feel any extended pain that keeps you from being able to relax.

If one of the needles continues to ache, pull, or throb uncomfortably for longer than one to five minutes, alert your practitioner to adjust the needle so that you are more comfortable.

Within seconds of all the needles being placed in your body, positive changes begin to take place. You can expect to feel immediately relaxed and calm. The breath begins to slow down and flow deeper down in the chest. Usually a sigh is released from deep in the abdomen, like an "ahhhh." We call that a "confirmation sigh," meaning the body is confirming that changes are beginning to take place. Often times, a stomach rumble or gurgling movement begins, which is another confirmation sign. This is your body responding to the Qi stimulus.

Usually within a few more minutes following insertion, my patients begin to experience a very deep and peaceful relaxation that allows for a meditative rest to emerge and take place in your body. It is almost as if the body and mind let go of all thoughts, worries, stress, and tightness. It's not because the needling part is over! Once your body connects with the altered electromagnetic currents, what I refer to as the "relaxation response" begins to kick in. Most or all negative energies are replaced with a meditative state of calmness;

your body may feel light and "floaty" (i.e., like you have had a couple of glasses of wine) or simply energized. Bodily tensions and pain usually subside during this time of quiet and rest, allowing the body's own "ecosystem" to achieve equilibrium. The streams within become clearer and cleaner; they have the enhanced ability to allow your body's energy, blood, and oxygen to move in a much more powerful and proficient manner.

By placing the needles accurately in the body, we can strengthen or tonify weaknesses, sedate excesses (where the body may be overstimulated), remove pain and muscular discomfort, warm or cool the body, or disperse stagnation or blocked Qi.

A treatment usually lasts from forty-five minutes to an hour after the needles have been placed in the body. It is just as likely that you will want to continue resting and choose to stay longer, if space and time allow. You may feel immediately rejuvenated and ready to go about your day. Many patients report feeling incredibly relaxed the day of a treatment, and on the following days, they feel revitalized and have more energy to tackle projects they have been putting off. In the best-case scenario, body pain or discomfort has begun to subside, although for some it may take a few more treatments. Most report increased mental clarity. Cravings for unhealthy food and other inappropriate substance choices are usually reduced.

The initial consultation can last anywhere from one and one-half to two hours because it includes not only your initial evaluation but also your first acupuncture treatment. After your first visit, it is best to schedule about one hour for further acupuncture appointments.

Refrain from getting an acupuncture treatment if you have been drinking, are drunk, or are taking recreational drugs. If you are taking pain medication for your symptoms, be sure to tell your practitioner. After your treatment, it is best to avoid exercise or strenuous athletics for twenty-four hours to allow the balancing that has taken place within the body to strengthen and take hold. It is also best to refrain from all forms of active sexual activity or orgasm for the first twenty-four hours after a treatment.

"My second baby was due in two weeks. My baby was in breech presentation, and my doctor wanted to schedule a C-section. I was completely against that idea and was frantic for alternatives. I was desperate to have a normal delivery, and when a friend recommended acupuncture, I decided to give it a try. During my acupuncture treatments, I could feel the baby turning inside of me. The treatments made me feel relaxed and rested. My baby boy was born in December, and although it was a hard labor, I was able to deliver vaginally. I am a believer in acupuncture now!"

—F.M., female, late thirties

INFORM

Chapter 6—Diet 101: Knowledge Is Power!

There is but one temple in the universe and that is the body of man.
—Novalis

We see in newspapers, magazines, and news reports and in our communities that we have a huge problem on our collective hands: obesity. Increasingly, we are finding ourselves more overweight than ever before in our society. We are slowly waking up and looking for change; we realize that we can no longer ignore our babies', our children's, our parents', and our own waistlines. This expansion puts us at risk for pain, disease, needless shame, and discomfort. But, when it comes to your diet, knowledge is the kind of power that can save your life.

Just like people have Qi, food also has its own Qi vibration. When we eat, we are consuming the enerQi of the food. It is very important to eat fresh fruits and vegetables, as they are alive with vitality. They carry with them a vibrant, clean energy from the yin of the earth and the yang of the sun. A diet of white flour and refined sugars does not have enough nourishment to keep you vital and glowing with powerful enerQi, as it lacks blood-producing nutrients. Remember, bagels alone do not a meal make!

Ideally, it is best to eat every three to four hours throughout the day to keep your enerQi and metabolism actively burning. Think of this method of eating as adding fuel to a burning fire. This method of eating can be thought of as the NONdiet. This is a healthy sensible way to enjoy a variety of food choices, never feel deprived, eat little bits of everything delicious, and still maintain a fit healthy physique!

Meal portions should not exceed the size of your palm. A small serving of protein, high-fiber foods, and a variety of fresh steamed seasonal vegetables, fresh fruits, nuts, or a garden salad make up most meals. Snacks can be six to eight almonds, a half a cup of yogurt, hummus on half a bagel or rice cake, a glass of fresh vegetable juice, or a small piece of fruit. Try almond butter on apple slices or celery, fresh fruit with nuts, dried fruits, string cheese, cottage cheese, yogurt, sliced turkey or chicken, fish, avocado, beans, fresh greens, and broth-based soups. These are all good foods that will fuel your body for activity throughout the day. The key to success is to be organized in your shopping and to have what you need on hand in your home or at your workplace. Another key is moderation and variety. There is no one-size-fits-all diet because we are all unique. I am not at all opposed to a vegetarian diet as long as the proper amounts of vegetable protein, fats, and carbohydrates are in balance.

As you learn to listen to your body, you will find that you eat when you are hungry and crave the foods that your body needs.

Fuel your body throughout the day by starting with breakfast. Oatmeal is an excellent choice because studies show that oats lower bad cholesterol (LDL) and slow the rise of blood glucose after eating. Eating oatmeal lowers your blood pressure, and the fiber leaves you feeling fuller for longer.

Foods takes on a different meaning as you naturally slow down and enjoy the tastes and the textures of the foods you are eating. You will also find that you are able to stop eating when you are satiated and before you are stuffed. Your next meal is coming right up when you are eating every three to four hours. Rather than eating gargantuan meals, become a healthy grazer! By eating every three hours, you will notice your energy, thinking, and emotions are more balanced throughout the day. People counterintuitively think that by not eating they will lose weight; however, not eating causes your metabolism to slow down to a crawl as it conserves calories to use as enerQi/fuel. By eating regularly, you will add enough fuel to power your body, and it will release fat stores. You will find that you will begin losing that extra weight you have been carrying around!

Pair a little bit of protein with your carbohydrates, and you will feel fuller longer.
Don't be afraid to add a little bit of "good" (unsaturated) fats to your diet. Fat in your diet does not equate to fat on your body. The right kinds of fats—unsaturated, omega-3 fats and olive oil—are essential brain food. They nourish the skin and hair, are vital anti-inflammatory/antiaging agents, and must not be eliminated from your diet.

Eating out is quite easy as most restaurants have a vegetable of the day, fresh salads, and a protein source. Being open to trying new foods and having variety in your diet is a good way to get out of a food rut. Once you open up to a new way of eating, most people really start to enjoy their new food life. It is important to think of these changes as permanent and positive lifestyle choices and not just another fad diet that is doomed to fail. This is a plan you can live with and love forever. Think of this as the "slow-the-aging-process inner power plan!" No one is 100 percent perfect, so when you do feel the need to splurge, enjoy it. Just start over as soon as possible on your healthy food path. With this attitude you will begin to feel much more in balance.

It's a good idea to eat fresh, in-season, preservative-free, or organic foods. Additionally, make sure that you wash all vegetables and fruits very well. As you get more accustomed to eating fresh fruits and vegetables, you will notice that every season has its own offering—eat those seasonal offerings whenever possible. By eating healthy foods, you supply clean, clear enerQi and sustenance to your body's vibrating root system. When you repeatedly make poor food choices, it is like pouring dirty water on a beautiful, vibrant plant. Remember, your body is your temple!

"I was a 340-pound overweight man with diabetes, high blood pressure, breathing problems, and sleep apnea. I was also very depressed. I had never tried acupuncture and was very skeptical. I was at a point, though, that something had to change, and I knew I needed help, or I was going to die. Through changes in my diet and lifestyle, along with weekly acupuncture and counseling sessions, I am proud to say that I have successfully lost 140 pounds. A new person has emerged from my old self! It has been a lot of hard work but an incredible journey. The acupuncture has helped me with my anxiety around life. I have been able to regain my energy, lower my blood pressure, and I can once again breathe without difficulty. My metabolism is able to work efficiently, and while I still have some work ahead of me, I couldn't have done it without my regular acupuncture treatments and the wisdom that Oriental medicine offers. Thank you for giving me back my life!"

—B.I., male, late forties

Chapter 7—Movement as Energy Exchange

When one must, one can.
—Yiddish proverb

One of the biggest challenges I see to the average individual coming into my clinic is lack of *intentional* exercise. Walking from the car in the parking lot to the store or restaurant is just not enough. You need at least 25 to 45 minutes of exercise three to five times a week, depending on your age and overall health.

Being outside, walking and breathing deeply, is a very good way to get the exercise you need. If winter conditions keep you inside, think about joining a gym or getting together with a friend at each other's homes to dance or do other forms of movement. Using videos is a great way to ensure a fun and interesting way of getting your exercise. There are so many choices available now; there really is a class or exercise right for everyone. Basically, make a commitment to get moving, period. Somehow, someway, do something that stretches and moves your body. Anything that will elevate your heart rate (within your own margins of safety) and that will cause your face to become lightly flushed will do the trick. It also helps to remember to maintain a pleasant expression throughout the experience. You have to be willing and ready to incorporate exercise into your life, and then it will become tolerable, if not fun. It is a gift you give to yourself. When energy moves, change becomes apparent almost immediately.

In the garden after the long cold winter, when it has been left untended, the soil is hard, with weeds popping up everywhere. You can't see the new, healthy, green growth; it's there, only obscured. When you begin working the soil a bit, pulling out weeds, watering, and fertilizing, new sprouts will begin to come up out of the ground. If you haven't tended your "garden" in a while, it is never too late to start. Think of your body as a garden, and begin your maintenance process. Nurture it and give it the care it needs to be strong and healthy for you!

Sexual health is also of great importance in moving and maintaining healthy Qi. Make the most of your experience—orgasms move energy and enhance your enerQi!

Stretching is another must. Flexibility is a very important component of fitness. It is vital that our tendons, ligaments, and important connective tissue remain supple as we age. It is paramount to the health and ease of movement within our bodies. With every stretch, you move the Qi, blood, and oxygen that nourishes and moistens your body's connective tissue that in turn supports your bones. Qi, blood, and oxygen cannot move freely to nourish our bodies if there is stagnation within the body.

In China, in the early morning hours, people from all walks of life are out in the parks doing tai chi and Qi gong (say "chee-gung") exercise. These exercises are designed to keep the body strong and supple, provide relaxation, and allow the mind to stay clear throughout the lifetime aging process. My master, Dr. Tan, practices regularly and teaches all his students and many of his patients Qi-building techniques that strengthen the mind and the body. Yoga is another great way to find your flexibility and relax your mind. Tai chi, Qi gong, and yoga all allow each of us to work at our own pace and achieve our own personal best. There is no competition!

"I have severe osteoarthritis in my left hip and moderate to severe osteoarthritis in my right hip, plus a bone spur in my left heel. My qualitative impression of acupuncture is that it seems to have arrested the deterioration at a minimum. I seem to walk with less of a limp than formerly. An unexpected side benefit is that I have also been able to lose thirty pounds that I was not able to shed previously. I have been receiving acupuncture treatments and nutritional counseling for more than six months now. The acupuncture sessions provide me with almost a trancelike-quality period of rest and rejuvenation, a feeling of overall well-being. The results have been wonderful in the context of my overall hectic personal and professional lifestyle. The respite is something that I look forward to every week, and the feeling of relaxation and well-being that it generates lasts especially throughout the day but also helps create a sense of greater calmness throughout the week. I benefit from my acupuncture treatments and always look forward to my visits/naps. Thank you for your help!"

—M.R., male, late sixties

Chapter 8—Sleep: There Is a Reason It's Called Beauty Rest

Too much of a good thing can be wonderful.
—Mae West

I often hear people say, "I will sleep when I die." It is an interesting saying because what people don't realize is that lack of sleep actually shortchanges their bodies of enerQi and vitality, making life a dull replica of what it can be. In fact, most people don't get enough sleep, even though 7 to 8 hours is the recommended daily dose. Your health and your ability to sleep restfully go hand in hand. Studies abound as to the benefits of sleep.

As we discussed earlier, our environment has its own energy vibration. Look around your bedroom; is it conducive to relaxation, sleep, and sexual intimacy? Are your bedroom and your life set up to provide the most beneficial sleeping experience? Bedrooms are best if they are painted in soothing shades. According to Chinese theory, colors representing passion and flesh colors are also good choices for the bedroom. If you can't control the color of the walls, choose accent pieces in shades of apricots, peaches, reds, pinks, and oranges (think evening sky at sunset). Light burgundies are an option but not too purple (purple often represents stagnation). Ideally, face your head to the north and your feet away from the door. When you walk into your bedroom, a feeling of peace and serenity should come over you as if you have just entered a relaxing spa or temple. If you must have a TV, avoid having it be the focal point of the room. Your bedroom is where you go to rest and recover from the rest of the world; make it reflect your idea of a sanctuary.

If you lie awake thinking and worrying, it is time to be honest about why. Are you worrying about money challenges? Do you live beyond your financial means? Is some aspect of your work unfulfilling or just no longer working for you? How are the relationships in your family? If you are with a significant other, do you feel safe and happy in that relationship? Whatever is on your mind, think about these issues outside of the bedroom so when you prepare for bed, you can let go mentally and relax.

Sleep allows your body, the engine that moves you around in your life, to shut down and regenerate. People who do not schedule enough time for sleep or who do not rest well when they do sleep, are more prone to anger, moodiness, depression, lack of patience, and indecision. Their minds are less sharp; they seem on edge and are often just not "with it." We have all seen examples of this type of person walking and, worse yet, driving around (it is not a pretty sight!). Over time, lack of sleep compromises your immune system, your thinking abilities, and your metabolism and speeds up the aging process.

Acupuncture alleviates sleep disorders, so if you have not had a treatment yet, this alone could be your answer to a good night's sleep. If you are experiencing dream-disturbed sleep on a regular basis, it might be a sign of unresolved emotional conflict. Often times, we emotionally process a lot of what goes on in our waking hours during our sleeping hours. If this is happening to you, it might be a sign to look at your life and make some changes. It is not uncommon to wake during the night to use the restroom and then go back to sleep. However, if you are having trouble getting back to sleep, tossing and turning, and watching minutes and hours tick away, you have a choice to continue and be frustrated and tired in the morning, or you can relax and meditate. By relaxing and breathing, you can shut down the mind and allow the body to let go of all tension.

Your mind can take you anywhere you let it. It can be hard to focus on finding that quiet place because the mind just will not turn off. This occurrence is referred to in Chinese medicine as "wondering mind." What can quiet the mind is meditation, and meditation is all about practice makes perfect.

First, create your own inner temple or sacred space by envisioning your perfect environment. For some, it helps to imagine a place in nature that calls to you: a beautiful ocean, a majestic mountain, flowing clear steams, cloud-filled skies, or rolling flower fields. If you are more kinesthetically inclined, holding on to an object such as a smooth gemstone or something that holds a special meaning to you can be quite calming. In this calm place, allow yourself to be free of distractions.

Then try this simple breathing exercise:
Begin by just closing your eyes. Relax the muscles around your eyes, in your face, and around your jaw. Relax your stomach, arms, hands, fingers, legs, feet, and toes. This feeling is akin to floating on a raft. Slightly open your jaw, and relax your mouth. Breathe slowly, feeling your breath begin to fill up your belly as if you were filling a beach ball. When you have filled up your belly to your point of comfort, using even slow breaths, exhale slowly and deeply, allowing your stomach and solar plexus to flatten. Inhale again, slowly filling up with your breath, filling that ball, and then exhale deeply. Allow all of this breathing action to happen in slow motion. With the inhalation, envision deep peace and serenity. With the exhalation, feel all tension leaving your body along with any fear, anxiety, sadness, and confusion.

Continue this breathing cycle until you feel yourself begin to relax from your head to your toes. You may find yourself drifting off to sleep, and that's OK. If you go back to your thoughts, allow yourself to just watch them float away like logs going down a stream. Using long and languid breaths, continue to deeply inhale and then deeply exhale. Soft music and hypnotherapy tapes are another great way to learn to relax and rest. Think of this practice as a higher mental training that must be mastered. Remember that the mind leads the Qi!

Dr. Tan once said this to me, and I have never forgotten it: "Life is an experience not unlike a huge roller coaster ride. There are great highs and long lows, but it is how one rides that is the key to happiness."

"After years of restless sleep, I was walking around exhausted, with true memory loss and impairment. My immune system was beginning to falter, and I was catching cold after cold. A friend of mine suggested I try acupuncture, and frankly, I was sick of taking nighttime sleep aids. This was not what nature intended! As I lay there during my first treatment, I was incredibly relaxed. I actually fell asleep on the table! I hadn't slept like that in years. As soon as Sheri put the needles in, it felt like a mild form of laughing gas from the dentist. By the time she closed the door, I was floating and on my way to a deep, relaxing nap. This relaxation stayed with me throughout the rest of the day; in fact, I was actually tired the rest of the evening and slept for five hours straight after my first treatment! I hadn't done that in years. After six months of treatments and herbal medication, I now enjoy a full night of rest every night. It has changed my life. No more colds! I can concentrate at work, and I am so much happier, just ask my husband!"

—A.L., forty-eight-year-old female

NATURAL

Chapter 9—Approach and Methods (Root and Branch)

Deep in their roots, all flowers keep the light.
—Theodore Roethke

In diagnosing one's internal medical challenges, Chinese medicine again draws from nature. We have all admired a great, majestic tree. Your health is like that great, majestic tree. The roots are your immune system, your Qi essence, and its power. The branches that shoot out from your tree are your subjective symptoms of a greater imbalance. The problem is not in the bad branch; it actually lies in the roots of the tree, the underlying cause of distress.

For example, I have a patient who suffered from terrible migraine headaches (branch). Rather than simply treat the headache, I looked at what else was going on within her ecosystem (e.g. the body) that could be the cause (the root) of the headache.

Patient A.G. is a very fit and physically active, forty-five-year-old female. She experienced migraines every month, lasting a week at a time, for fifteen years. She slept terribly and reported anxiety over the same time frame. She also complained of poor digestion and ongoing fatigue.

In considering the root and branch theory, I know that the headaches are a symptom and not the cause of dysfunction. Using acupuncture and herbs, I was able to get her sleeping soundly for 6 to eight hours a night. That alone decreased her anxiety level, and she was, under her doctor's and my supervision, slowly able to wean herself off of her antianxiety medication and sleeping pills. I analyzed her nutrition and put her on a program that included more warm vegetables, nourishing soups, and less cold salads. The warmth activates the spleen and encourages and initiates better digestion and elimination. Once her sleep, anxiety, and digestion became more in balance, her hormones adjusted as well. Her ongoing fatigue started to improve once she was digesting better because she was able to get more nutrition from better food choices. The quality of her sleep was much more sound because she had less stomach distress, which had been contributing to keeping her up and uncomfortable. Voila! Fewer headaches within one menstrual cycle!

I have been treating this patient for six months now and she has experienced almost a complete cessation of migraines. We still have more work to do in balancing out her body, but we are more than halfway there.

I always listen very carefully to what my patients' "chief complaint" is; however, I am always exploring the deeper levels to uncover what is truly causing their imbalance.

The "root and branch" diagnostic theory dictates from within you where we need to begin to balance and correct the disharmony. This means that your condition is not the cause of the dis-ease; it is merely the manifestation or branches of the true, underlying root cause, with the exception of a sports injury, sprain, or strain. If only symptoms are treated and the fundamental root cause is not addressed, it is like constantly bailing water out of a leaking boat rather then fixing the leak in the first place.

"I first discovered acupuncture in February 1998. I was desperate. I couldn't work for six months due to extreme muscle weakness, aches, dizziness, and stiffness in my joints. I had lost fifteen pounds and couldn't gain weight no matter what I ate. I had erratic menstrual cycles and loose bowels. I had been to several doctors, and every test turned out negative. I had been told by a couple of doctors that I had chronic fatigue syndrome and that there was nothing they could do. I was resigned to the fact that I would probably be this way the rest of my life because all the literature on the topic was doom and gloom.

Through a friend, I found acupuncture. I was assured that I could be helped, which was a shock to me, especially after all those months of doctors telling me nothing could be done. I was scared but decided to try it. My stiffness noticeably improved after my very first visit. My prescription was twice a week treatments of acupuncture for several months, dietary modifications, and herbal medicines. Within three months, I was back to work, albeit on a shortened schedule. It took about a year for a complete recovery. As I continued with my treatments, I was able to look at my life differently. Not only did I regain my strength, I found a new confidence and felt more in control of my life. I am now more patient with others and myself. I have changed my diet and am healthier, mentally and physically. Acupuncture literally gave me my life back!"

—A.L.C., forty-three-year-old female

Chapter 10—The Elements Within: A Deeper Understanding of Diagnosis

A man is what he wills himself to be.
—Jean Paul Sartre

The elements of nature that Oriental medicine assigns to our pulses are the same ones used to explain the way our body functions. The elements of Fire, Earth, Metal, Water, and Wood symbolize the interrelationships of organs. We call this order of elements the "control and nourish cycle." As you're reading about the elements and body functions, keep in mind that the Oriental concepts of body functions and organ systems are different from the Western way of thinking. Acupuncturists take Western concepts into consideration but expand on them. For example, when I say "liver," remember that I'm not only speaking of the liver's functions of cleansing blood and digesting nutrients; in Oriental medicine, the liver's functions are more encompassing.

An example of how the elements are used in diagnosis can be found in the concept of the twelve pulses and their relationship to one another. These relationships are interdependent, as each one feeds another. To understand the control and nourish cycle, let's return to the analogies of nature by again picturing a great, strong tree planted in the earth. This tree gets much-needed energy to grow and thrive from the warmth of the sun and the quality of the soil. The soil also feeds the roots so they can spread freely. The water from the rain and snow nourish and moisten these roots, which enable the trunk, bark, and branches to grow strong and continue to flourish. This cycle continues year after year, drawing upon and feeding upon these important elements in nature. Each of these elements depends on and assists others to nurture and grow. This cooperation of elements allows for healthy Qi and sustained longevity.

Fire, Earth, Metal, Water, and Wood exist in our material world. Each element carries within it its own yin/yang energy. The elements can function alone but work best if they act together. These elements depend, assist, act, and counteract upon one another. Because these elements need one another to function, if out of balance, one can cause another to malfunction.

These elements, like life itself, are in constant motion, are cyclical, and are always changing. We assign elements to our internal organs, outward extremities, and psychological and emotional states. Each element, along with its associated organs, has a specific time of day or night for optimal functioning. This time element serves as a check and balance system within the body. These elements help to paint an archetype of thought, word, and deed for the doctor who is using all of his or her senses to make accurate diagnoses. These archetypes are broad generalizations based on the characteristics of each element. Most people will have a true dominant element and one or two secondary elements that are active within the body at the same time. Read the following descriptions, and you may begin to see yourself, or someone close to you, functioning within these concepts.

Fire Attributes

The organs of the Fire element are the heart (yin), which is at its peak between 11:00 AM and 1:00 PM, and the small intestine (yang), which peaks between 1:00 PM and 3:00 PM. The Fire element is known as the king because the heart pumps blood through the vessels to the entire body. The heart contains the spirit, also known as *shen*, which houses and controls the mind. The small intestine plays a role in the body's water distribution process and metabolism. The small intestine separates the impure waste materials from the pure nutritious elements of foods. The pure elements are circulated throughout the body, and the impure elements are sent on to the large intestine which is known as the receiver.

You are directly experiencing the heart element when you are feeling happiness, laughing, or hearing the sound of laughter. The Fire season is the summer, the direction is south, the color is red or pink, the taste is bitter, and the smell is scorched or burnt. The tongue is the flower of the heart; this means the tongue, especially the tip, can tell me the condition of a patient's heart element. For example, if you came to me with sores on your tongue, it would be a tip-off for me to pay attention to the heart element.

Fire personalities have an intimate, warm, open, expressive, and compassionate temperament. Their facial colors tend toward redness or a white gray; their walk is bouncy and fast. The head or chin will often be pointed, and they tend to have smaller hands. Their hair is usually curly or sparse. They can be active, energetic, smart, inventive, alert, and excitable, yet sometimes scattered. Fire types appreciate beauty, can have explosive tempers, and are prone to chaos (think of a firecracker going off with many colors filling the sky all at once). Fire types are typically great talkers, crave spicy hot foods (fire feeds fire), tend toward nervousness, and love fame and recognition. When there is an imbalance, they can become overly talkative, often missing social cues to stop and listen. This could be an indication of "shen" disturbance.

An excess in the Fire element sometimes manifests as dizziness, a urinary tract infection, heart palpitation, or angina. Typically, there is sleep disturbance or dream-disturbed sleep. Inappropriate laughter is common, as well as prolonged emotional sadness or mental illness. Excessive walking strains the Fire element (i.e., walking for hours on end).

Earth Attributes

The organs of the Earth element are the spleen (yin), which is at its peak between 9:00 AM and 11:00 AM, and the stomach (yang), which peaks between 7:00 AM and 9:00 AM. The spleen and the stomach are the main organs of digestion and assimilate food and fluids. These organs are collectively referred to as the "center" of the body. The spleen regulates the blood and helps to keep it within the channels. It transforms food into nourishment and moves those nutrients upward to the stomach. The stomach regulates the sea of nourishment, performing the "rottening and ripening" process as it receives the food and moves nutrients downward. The Earth element houses the thoughts and controls the flesh and the limbs. The mouth is the flower of the spleen and stomach.

The Earth's direction is the center, and its smell is of sweetness and perfume. The emotion is pensiveness or deep thinking; the sound is of singing. You are directly experiencing the energy of the Earth element when you taste sweetness, when you wear the colors orange, yellow, beige, or brown, or when you enjoy the end days of summer.

Earth types are relaxed, slow, sensitive, and sweet. They love pleasure, and are generous, kind, calm, and can be overly sensitive. Typically, but not always, the stomach can be chunky and large, with a soft belly. The head and jaw is often large and wide. Earth types have softer, cuddly flesh, yet are full and muscular. The upper arm skin sometimes hangs below the muscle. When they walk, they do not lift their feet very high (grounded to the Earth). Earth types love to save, save, save, and they are often referred to as "pack rats." They tend to love the simple things in life and are not overly ambitious. They are deep thinkers who tend to chew their cud (mental ruminators). They always want more, especially sugary sweets.

You can tell when an Earth type is out of balance because they seem scattered with confused thinking. They may have difficulty concentrating, often forgetting what they were doing or where they were going in the first place. A deficiency in the Earth element weakens the spleen, causing dampness, indigestion, bloating, and tiredness after meals. In contrast, dryness weakens the stomach, which manifests as acid indigestion, ulcers, pain, or burning. Most deficient disorders in the body's center stem from the spleen; most excess disorders in the body's center stem from the stomach. Excess sitting strains the Earth element. When the spleen is weak, the body is unable to use the nutrients from food. Often, this is due to a surplus of iced or cold foods and beverages or overly spicy foods. This challenge can be corrected with a change of diet, which would include more appropriate food choices. Excessive worry injures and weakens the Earth element.

Metal Attributes

The organs of the Metal element are the lungs (yin), which peak between 3:00 AM and 5:00 AM, and the large intestine (yang), which peaks from 5:00 AM to 7:00 AM. The Metal element is known as the prime minister because it is in charge of the orderly rhythm of Qi and breath in the body. The lungs are responsible for breathing and take in the Qi from the air while governing the Qi or energy states within the body. The lungs are the master of Qi and govern the voice and the skin. The lungs house what is referred to as the "corporeal soul," which is the physical part of the soul that manifests as feelings and sensations. The corporeal soul is linked to our breath and our ability to take long, deep, open, cleansing breaths.

The large intestine is called the "Official of Transport" and is responsible for elimination. It extracts water from the impure essence it receives from the small intestine, transports the liquid waste to the bladder, and excretes the solid leftover waste as stool. Those who are experiencing the energy of the metal element will often feel emotionally wistful. The Metal sound is crying or whining; the season is autumn. The Metal direction is west, the color is metallic or white, the taste is pungent or spicy, and the smell is fishy or rank. The nose is the flower of the lungs.

A Metal personality reflects the traits of a temperament that is often inspired, courteous, disciplined, refined, precise, formal, and happy after accomplishments. It is quite common for Metal types to well up while watching a movie trailer or hearing a sad story. This is a reflection of their sensitive souls. They are typically fine featured with small bones yet have broad, strongly built bodies and square shoulders. They tend to walk slowly and deliberately and will sometimes have a strong voice. Their health is reflected in the skin and hair (think shiny and bouncy), although they sometimes have a tendency toward dryness. Metal types can be strict with themselves and others, are attached to their ideas, can be neurotic, and will not stop at a task until it is their idea of perfection, as they have strong wills. Too much talking weakens the Metal element, as does excessive grief and melancholy.

A deficiency in the Metal element often manifests as an inability to take deep, long breaths. Lung types are often uncomfortable with and have difficulty expressing feelings. Their corporeal soul becomes weak because of an inability to take those deep, cleansing breaths. Many Metal types report tightness in the chest, asthma, and a compromised immune system. The lungs are the most delicate of the organs and are the first to be attacked by external evil pathogens (common colds and flus) when the body is weak. Rashes are common as the lungs control the metabolism within the body that distributes liquid to bathe and moisten the skin.

Water attributes

The organs of the Water element are the kidneys (yin), which are at their peak from 5:00 PM to 7:00 PM, and the urinary bladder (yang), which peaks from 3:00 PM to 5:00 PM. The kidneys are responsible for reproduction, growth, and regeneration. They are said to be the ministers of health because of the importance of their role. The bladder is called the outlying district official; it controls and transports the body's fluids and excretes them. The kidneys are the gate of vitality, which is *very* important, as this is the source of the body's enerQi and power for all the internal organs. Diagnosis *always* takes into consideration the health of the kidneys because they are the root of yin and yang in the body. The kidneys house our willpower. They also house the "Ming Men Fire" known as the "Gate of Vitality." The most important job of the Gate of Vitality energy force is that it creates heat/fire, which creates movement of energy, and therefore creates power within us, like an engine. Ming Men Fire heats our body and allows the kidney essence to have the power to perform daily tasks needed for proper body functioning. For this reason, the kidneys are called the battery pack of the body.

You are experiencing the Water element when you feel fear or hear the sounds of tiresome groaning and grumbling. The season and climate is winter and cold. The Water direction is north, the color is black, purple, or blue, the taste is salty, and the smell is rotten or putrid. The ears are the flower of the kidneys, while the openings are the urethra and the anus.

A Water type's temperament is easygoing, calm, creative, willful, ambitious, sensitive, sympathetic, and sometimes psychic. They are perceptive, aware, sharp thinking, loyal to friends, eccentric, and flexible in their personalities. They can eat most things because they typically have a strong digestive system. Water element types swing when walking and flow like waves. They can have a round face and body, with soft, pale, lighter skin or have red flushed cheeks with more of a thin, wiry frame. Typically, this type has difficulty holding on to body weight even though they are good eaters who are always grazing on food and snacks throughout the day and night.

Water types can be jumpy or quick to startle yet love to lie about and lounge. They are prone to telling little white lies. The reflection of strong health within the Water element can be found in the condition of the bones, marrow, brain, hair (premature graying and hair loss), teeth, inner ear, pupils, and lumbar region, which houses the kidney essence.

Overexposure to fright or fear weakens the Water element. A deficiency in the Water element can manifest as high- or low-frequency ear ringing, infertility, low back pain, weak vision, confusion, apathy, and sorrow. If imbalanced, Water types can run a very hot body temperature, with sweaty palms. They can become so hyper that they can't rest when they lie down and often have night sweats with restless sleeping. With deficiency, they can be clammy or chilly and will want to lie shivering in a curled fetal position, trying to get warm. A kidney weakness will always show up as dark or gray circles under the eyes. With this weakness comes the need for a lot of rest because they tire easily and have since childhood. Children will often fail to thrive and have higher incidences of asthma.

Any chronic condition will always involve the kidneys; your practitioner will seek to maintain the strength and vitality of the kidneys with every treatment. A lifestyle of excess will strain the Water element. Exhaustion, excessive sexual activities, over exercise, long periods of standing, excessive drinking, and external attacks of cold (catching a chill) are common causes of long-term weakness. Women often have weak or no menstruation, and men often moan and groan in frustration about impotence, weak sex drive, or premature ejaculation. Both will have frequent occurrences of urination, especially at night. Chronic low back pain is common.

Wood attributes

The organs of the Wood element are the liver (yin), which is at its peak between 1:00 AM and 3:00 AM, and the gallbladder (yang), which peaks from 11:00 PM and 1:00 AM. The liver is said to be the general within the body as its function is one of planning, organizing, and coordination between the organs. The liver stores the blood and regulates the movement and flow of Qi within the body. It regulates the other organs because of its function of spreading Qi. It houses "the ethereal soul," which is said to influence our sense of direction in life, our emotions, and our capacity to plan our life's pursuits. Another important function of the liver is to nourish and bathe the tendons, ligaments, muscles, and joints with moisture, allowing for suppleness and flexibility. The gallbladder is named the judge because it is responsible for decision making. The gallbladder stores and secretes bile, which is produced by the liver. It is said to purify yang energy, holding the pure and impure essence of the body.

It can be said that you are experiencing the Wood element when you feel anger or frustration, shout or hear shouting, and enjoy the season of spring. The Wood climate is windy, the direction is east, the color is green or blue green, the taste is sour, and the smell is yeasty or damp. The eyes are the flower of the liver and, with the nails, reflect the health of the liver.

Wood personalities are hard working, talkative, confident, competitive, and bold achievers who are precise. A lot of Wood element body types are thin, wiry, and compact, with firm, tight muscles, or they can be quite muscular and strong, with broad shoulders. In excess, they are easily irritated and prone to anger, moodiness, and temperamental behaviors, such as temper tantrums and yelling. They are known to be self-important. This behavior is referred to as being "liverish," and is very easy to spot. They are the bores in restaurants who yell at the staff for forgetting their waters! They have a tendency to worry, find it hard to relax, and can be prone to depression. Meditation, yoga, having lots of fun, and staying up into the wee hours of the morning are what make a Wood element personality happy. Most Wood element people characterize themselves as "night owls," although they really need to be in bed by 11:00 PM. Otherwise, they get an energetic second wind and will happily be up until 2:00 AM because the liver is regenerating during this time.

Those with Wood disharmony always are attracted to and love the color purple. They wear it often (yes, to the clinic for treatments) and are known to even paint their homes in various shades of purple. Depression and anger disturb the quality of Wood's functioning, which is free flowing. Interestingly, the Chinese character for the liver signifies flowing and free. Many women suffer from liver Qi disharmony (stagnation) because its function is so closely related to the storage of blood; hence its connection to PMS. Excessive reading strains the liver; walking is the exercise of the liver. When there is a weakness in the gallbladder, there will often be indecision and timidity. Deficient Wood types will have trouble deciding what to wear, what to eat, what to do, where to go, or even if they should bother to go at all.

When the Wood element is imbalanced, it is common to see neck and shoulder tension, headaches, high blood pressure, gas, stomach cramps, or a very tight stomach with nausea (before, during, and after eating). A sensation like a pit in the throat is often felt (this is called plum pit Qi). Urinary tract infections are common. Yellowish eyes, uncontrolled shaking, or restless leg syndrome are sometimes present. With wood imbalance, it is not uncommon for patients to be diagnosed with Bells palsy and other neuralgias.

As you can see, there is a very strong and vital yin/yang relationship within each of the organs. One cannot function without the help of the other. The temperatures within these elements vary based on excess or deficiency, manifesting their balance or imbalance as wind, dampness, dryness, heat, or cold. Temperatures are important to take into consideration when diagnosing and treating.

You will be able to identify a small part of yourself in each of the elemental characterizations. A good practitioner is able to ascertain which parts of these characterizations make up the most of who you are and work from there to create balance and harmony.

Below is a condensed chart of these elements to give you a better idea of these concepts.

Keeping in mind the cycle of life, the ancient texts say:

- Fire renews the Earth and is extinguished by Water.
- Earth creates Metal and is penetrated by Wood.
- Metal holds Water and is melted by Fire.

- Water nurtures Wood and is contained by Earth.
- Wood feeds Fire and is cut by Metal.

At age thirty-six, shortly after my first and only pregnancy, I developed exercise-induced asthma that quickly worsened. It seemed that everything and nothing exacerbated my symptoms. Worse yet, the medications I was prescribed caused miserable side effects. While taking inhaled steroids and [allergy medication], I experienced cloudy thinking, blurred vision, disturbed sleep patterns, and anxiety. The treatment was as bad as the disease, which continued to worsen. I had never known anyone who received acupuncture other than an acquaintance receiving treatment for hormonal problems. Out of desperation I decided to try acupuncture, although this was a very different path than the one I followed as an educated professional with a bachelor of science in nursing and a law degree. I was not so much skeptical as I was uninformed.

Within three months, I had stopped taking the inhaled steroids and the [allergy medication]. Within one year, I noticed that I was back to using my inhaled [steroids] only prior to exercise and not with every change in the weather and every single viral illness. Further, I was overjoyed at the unintended—for me—benefits of acupuncture. My atypical, atopic dermatitis, present for over ten years, had lessened in severity. The mood swings and many other physical symptoms I experienced as a result of early menopause were muted. I was sleeping more deeply and restfully, even though I had been a lifelong insomniac.

There are many illnesses, syndromes, and conditions that I now know, as a result of personal experience as well as reading and research, are helped by acupuncture. It is a real therapy that made a real difference in my life and has helped me to gain a higher level of health and well-being.

—R.H., female, midforties

ENERGY

Chapter 11—The Mind Leads the Qi: It's an Inside Job

He who cannot change the very fabric of his thought will never be able to change reality, and will never, therefore, make any progress.

—Anwar Sadat

The mind leads the Qi. Your mind acts as the master and your Qi as the servant. By shifting your thoughts, your energetic frequency is elevated to a much higher level. As you fine-tune your body's Qi voltage, you will notice that you attract positive changes in your life and your health.

Once again, think of your body as a pathway, a stream, that carries your own channel of energy fields. Your thoughts start the chain of command, the beginning of your Qi stream. Qi begins in your mind and takes direction from your thoughts that instruct it to flow along the pathways into your body. This is typically an unconscious process; however, if your thoughts are toxic (and we all know what that means!), it is the perfect breeding ground for disease and distress.

Your emotions, negative or positive thinking, direct your Qi along the meridians in your body like water down a stream. The consequences of negative thinking, poor lifestyle choices, and lack of coping mechanisms lead to a compromised and weakened immune system, which makes us all susceptible to sickness and disease. Lifestyle choices include the things we choose to eat, the exercise we get or don't get, the amount of alcohol or drugs (prescription or recreational) we use, the amount of sleep we get, and how we take care of ourselves emotionally.

Your thoughts work like magnets; what you are thinking you will create and attract energetically. What you think, what you say, and how you say it are other forms of conscious powerful attraction. As you experience natural positive electromagnetic energy, you will find it easier and easier to visualize yourself achieving what you want in life, whether it is your ideal relationship, shape, weight, job, or fitness level. With regular practice, it gets easier to see in your mind's eye a healthy, happy, glowing, and relaxed person. This is the "YOU" you want to see yourself as, the "YOU" you will create for yourself. If you are having trouble seeing yourself in this way, imagine you are talking to a trusted friend or caring for a treasured animal you love very much. What would you say to him if he were not well and obviously "out of balance"? What would you want for him? How would you get him the help he needs to get to his ideal place of wellness? When you come up with the answers, put your ideas into action. Start your mental chain of Qi moving in a changed direction. You will make that new thought become reality. It really is an inside job. You create wellness with your enerQi.

Allow yourself to go on a positive thinking and speaking diet. If a thought comes into your head that is anything but positive or empowering, send it away immediately. If it doesn't feel good to think about or say, chances are it is not good for you or anyone else. Learn to monitor your thoughts. Watch your thoughts flow into the field of your mind. Identify what kind of thought you are having. Are they positive and constructive or negative and destructive? Practice mind control and consciously choose only thoughts that serve you and others in a positive way. If what you are thinking does not enhance your life or the lives of others, toss those thoughts away like a log that rushes down the river. You can choose to do this simply because you say so. It all starts in your mind.

"I first tried acupuncture because I am a runner and was experiencing pain in my hip. My GP examined me, took x-rays and said he couldn't find anything wrong with me, but if it hurt, to stop running (not an option, if you know runners!). I tried chiropractic, with mixed results. After running through the pain for almost two years, I was open to try anything but surgery or drugs. Oriental medicine was a welcome and pleasant surprise, because I was treated as a whole person not as a specific injury. Not only was my hip pain cured, I noticed that with treatments and a few tweaks of my lifestyle choices I no longer got cold sores and avoided the fatigue that I fought valiantly for years with caffeine. I found that I was totally chilled out after treatments and a lot less irritated by the little things and people in life. I am now hooked and know when I need to go in for my "attitude adjustment"!

—T.A.S., 29-year-old female

Chapter 12—On Becoming More Round

As we express our gratitude, we must never forget that the highest appreciation is not to utter words, but to live by them.
—John F. Kennedy

You may be asking yourself, "What does it mean to 'become more round'?" Chinese philosophy regarding energy is that we operate in a constant shifting of movement between yin and yang, or heaven and earth. When you look at the symbol for yin and yang, one of the first things to notice is that it is round with two symbols enclosed within it. There are no sharp edges or angles; everything flows around the yin and yang symbol. Each half blends and gives way to the other. They depend on one another for balance, harmony, and wholeness. Each contains a round circle of the opposite color, representing the opposite energy within its center. Because they are interdependent, they are conduits of energy for each other and themselves. You could say they feed off each other's actions and reactions.

So, how does the concept of yin and yang translate into our everyday world? The decisions we make every day influence this delicate balance of our enerQi. As we discussed earlier, everything from what we eat to how much we sleep and from how much activity we get to the positive or negative interactions we have with others directly impacts our enerQi. Knowing this, we must consciously make new decisions that balance us. Some of these decisions can involve relationships within our communities. We can see the nature of balance and imbalance when we observe the circumstances that unfold in our lives because of our actions. Some may say, "We reap what we sow"; others call it karma. We may not like the messages we are getting from life when things aren't going our way. However, rather than feel indignant, take it is an opportunity to look for the message and ask, "What actions am I taking that warrant this?" and "What seeds am I sowing, and how can I change my fate?"

Many people operate from a mindset of, "What's in it for me?" that emphasizes receiving. While it is important to take care of yourself and those you love, we do not live in a vacuum. We are all interconnected, and our actions and decisions affect those around us. Giving to others—loved ones, your community, even strangers—serves as a counterweight to receiving and balances us. This type of giving back increases our dimensions, rounds us out, and opens us up in a grander sense. It is not just about writing a check to an important cause (although that is a great way to give and is much needed in our world). This giving back encompasses the actions of donating yourself, your time, your wisdom, and your presence to a cause or individual. It can be as simple as asking a store clerk how his day is going and maintaining eye contact while waiting to hear his response. It is holding the elevator door for someone that is running to catch it. Consciously, you step out of yourself and into someone else's world. It is the time spent volunteering to help others in need.

It is the random acts of kindness that indeed do come back to us and make the world a better place for all. We have all had the experience in our daily lives of someone cutting us off or being rude to us, and the interaction stays with us for moments, hours, or even days. It affects the enerQi of our spirit and can affect our interactions with other people if we allow it to. Energy attracts its own type of energy; like attracts like, so be mindful of the kind of energy you are putting out there! As we embrace the principles of energy and balance in our lives, you might consider and participate in the concept of giving back. You will find that when you are in tune, everything seems to fall into place effortlessly.

By stepping out of ourselves and into our communities, we are able to maintain another type of balance between the world of others and ourselves. We all have a gift, a special skill or knowledge in our field, or a deeper wisdom we can share with the world. Perhaps you can donate your time and become a Big Brother or Big Sister, read to the elderly in nursing homes, or plant trees in your community. The opportunities and ideas to give back are endless. As you give back, in small ways and in big ways, you will observe a shift in what you receive. Things flow into place for you as both you and the world become more balanced between giving and receiving. As more and more people catch on, these actions will start to become normal behaviors for us all. A domino effect will begin to occur. Your actions will cause reactions; a veritable ripple effect through society will happen. Like the yin/yang symbol, all good deeds flow back to the source; the cycle continues.

It's hard to believe that it has only been a year since I walked into your office, all 108 pounds of me on a five-feet-ten-inch frame! Six months prior, I had left a treatment facility for anorexia and could feel myself losing weight again. I was very afraid and knew I needed help. With acupuncture, I started to sleep again and my anxiety levels were greatly diminished. I started to see my life and myself differently. I began gaining weight and felt healthy about it. I have now gained twenty-five pounds and feel so grateful to finally be at a different place in my life. I had always wondered what people meant when they talked about being "balanced." Now I know it's not some "new age" term. It is a really wonderful feeling. Acupuncture saved my life! Thank you!

—J.A., female, late twenties

Chapter 13—Your New Beginning

Life can be, if you allow it, like a roller coaster ride: up one day down the next. Act from your inner center. Whether things go well for you or ill, reflect: All things must change. Don't get elated or depressed, for nothing in this universe will remain the same forever. Practice even mindedness.

—Anonymous

So there you have it. The LAINE method! Learn. Align. Inform. Natural. Energy. A powerful concept of balance in Oriental medicine. Acupuncture serves to balance yin and yang, oxygenate your blood, enhance your energy, fuel your metabolism, and lift your mind. The delicate balance between yin and yang is affected by your daily choices: what you eat, how much you sleep, how much exercise or movement you incorporate into your day, your outlook on life, as well as the people and environment you surround yourself with. As you become more balanced, you will discover that it is easier to sense when you are off balance.

By tuning into yourself and your life, you will be empowered to make stronger, healthier, and more powerful decisions. It is just a given: when your enerQi is vibrating with a strong electromagnetic current, you will see that you attract like energies to yourself. Your thoughts are big magnets that become your reality. You will discover as you begin to live a more balanced life that you are creating and experiencing more joy, laughter, love, and happiness in all areas of your life. It is a central law of the universal energetic flow. We create with our thoughts and our energetic vibration.

Life abounds with possibility and is full of a myriad of choices. You have the unique opportunity and position to choose the life you want to lead and the power to make the decisions to take you where you want to go. With that power comes the ability to make educated health choices that honor and support your body. Walking down a different path may feel uncomfortable or foreign at first because it is new to you. With an open mind, you always have the reassurance of going back to where you were. But then again, you may just never want to look back! Welcome to your new beginning.

Majestic trees
Alive with abundance
Like your body, heavenly
SL

978-0-595-41555-7
0-595-41555-5

Printed in the United States
64891LVS00001B/73-96

9 780595 415557